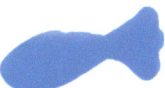

For my husband Mark, who helps make my dreams come true.

For our children Ayden, London, Brie and Cohen,
My biggest dream was you.

For Jonathan and Michelle Giles for never giving up on me
even though I tend to do things the hard way.

For all of the friends and family who told me this
dream would come true someday.

Printed in the United States of America

First Printing, 2022

Xan Pulsipher | Established 2022 | USA

All Clammed Up

by Xan Pulsipher

illustrated by Victoria Arvidson

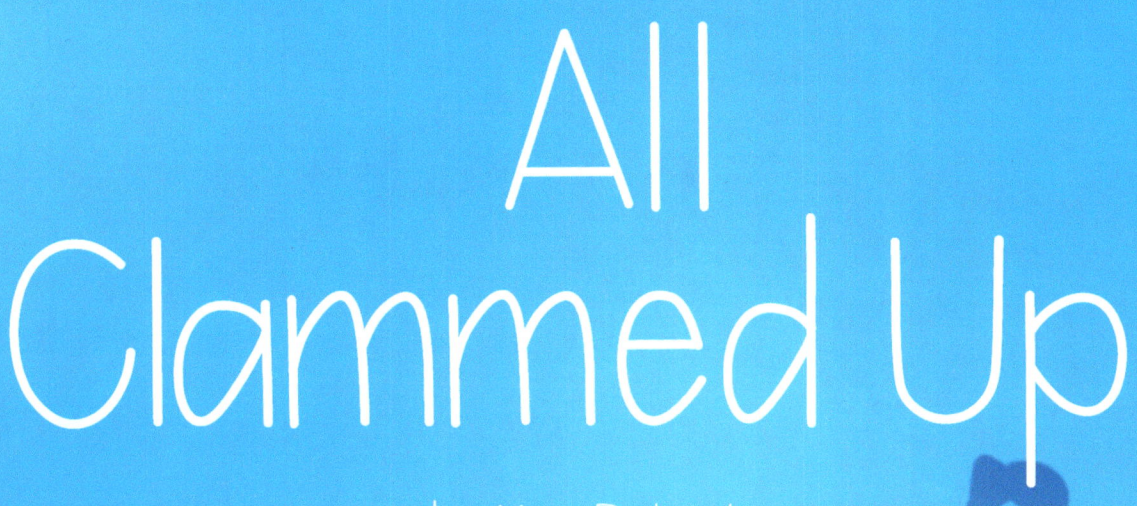

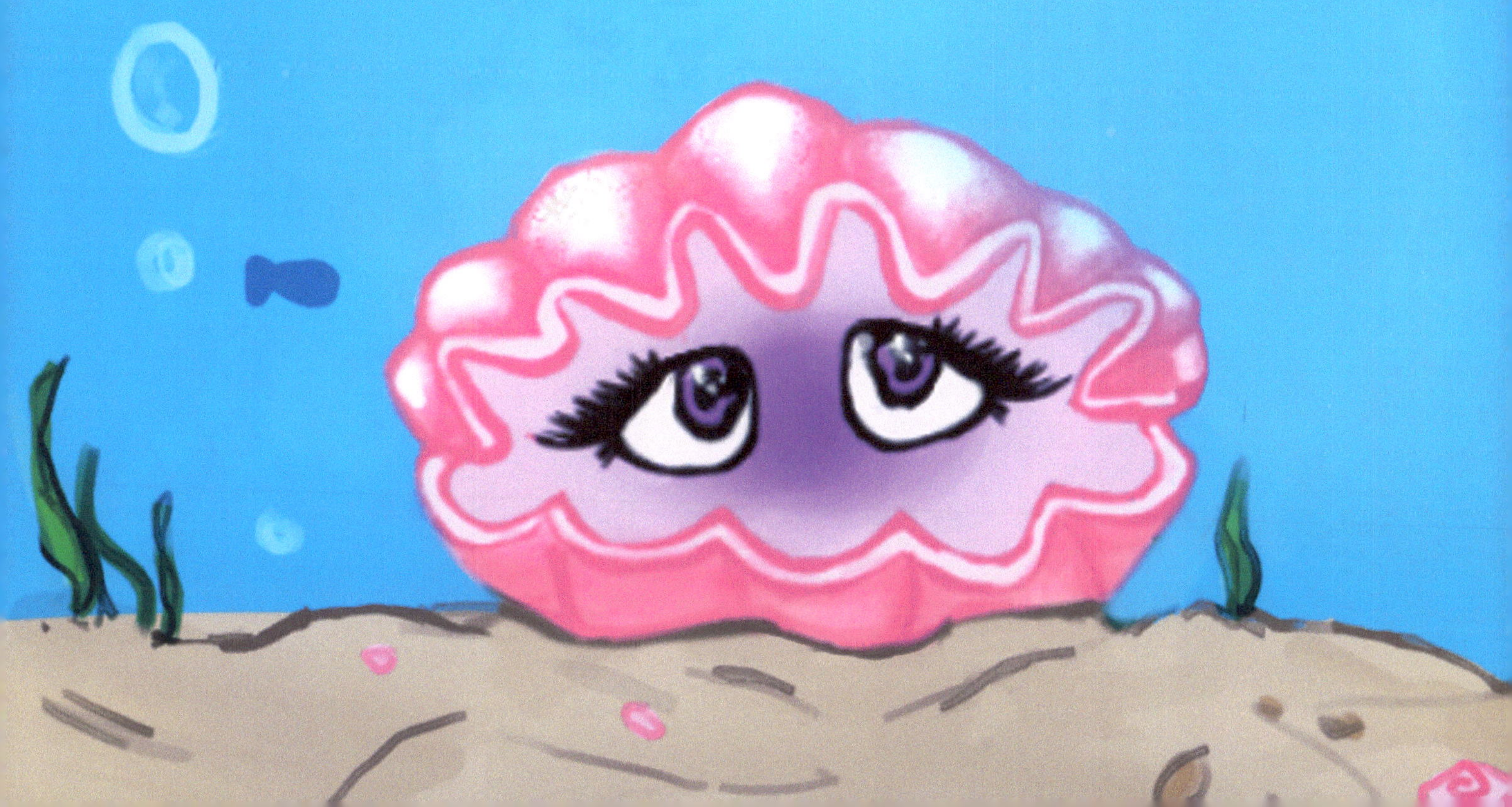

Chloe the Clam sat sadly upon the silent sea floor,
Staring up at the creatures above her, she wished she was more.
She watched them in envy, their lives so exciting and free,
Were so much better, than hers could ever be.
"What a lonely life I live laying here on the bottom of the sea.
Look at how amazing they are! They are all so much better than me."

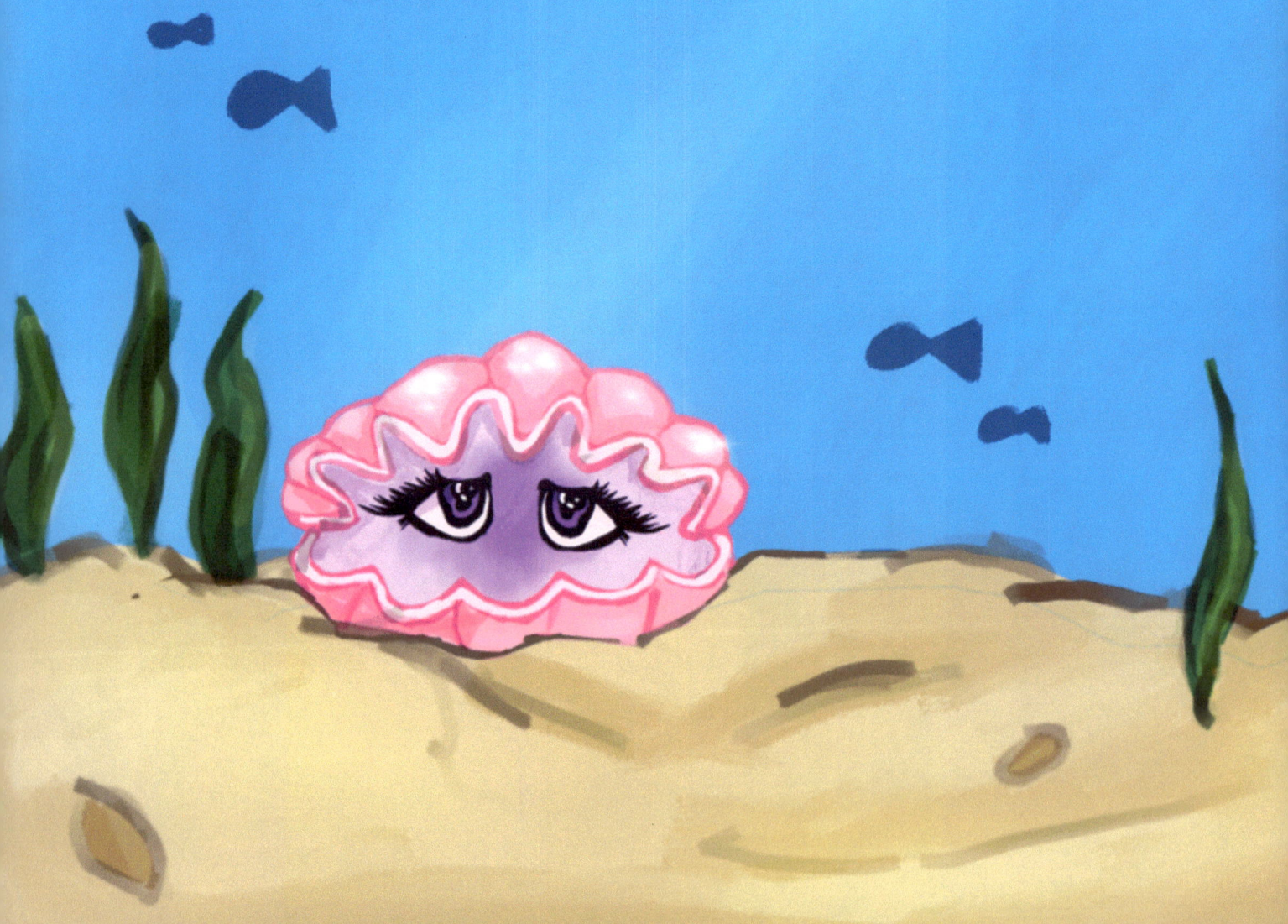

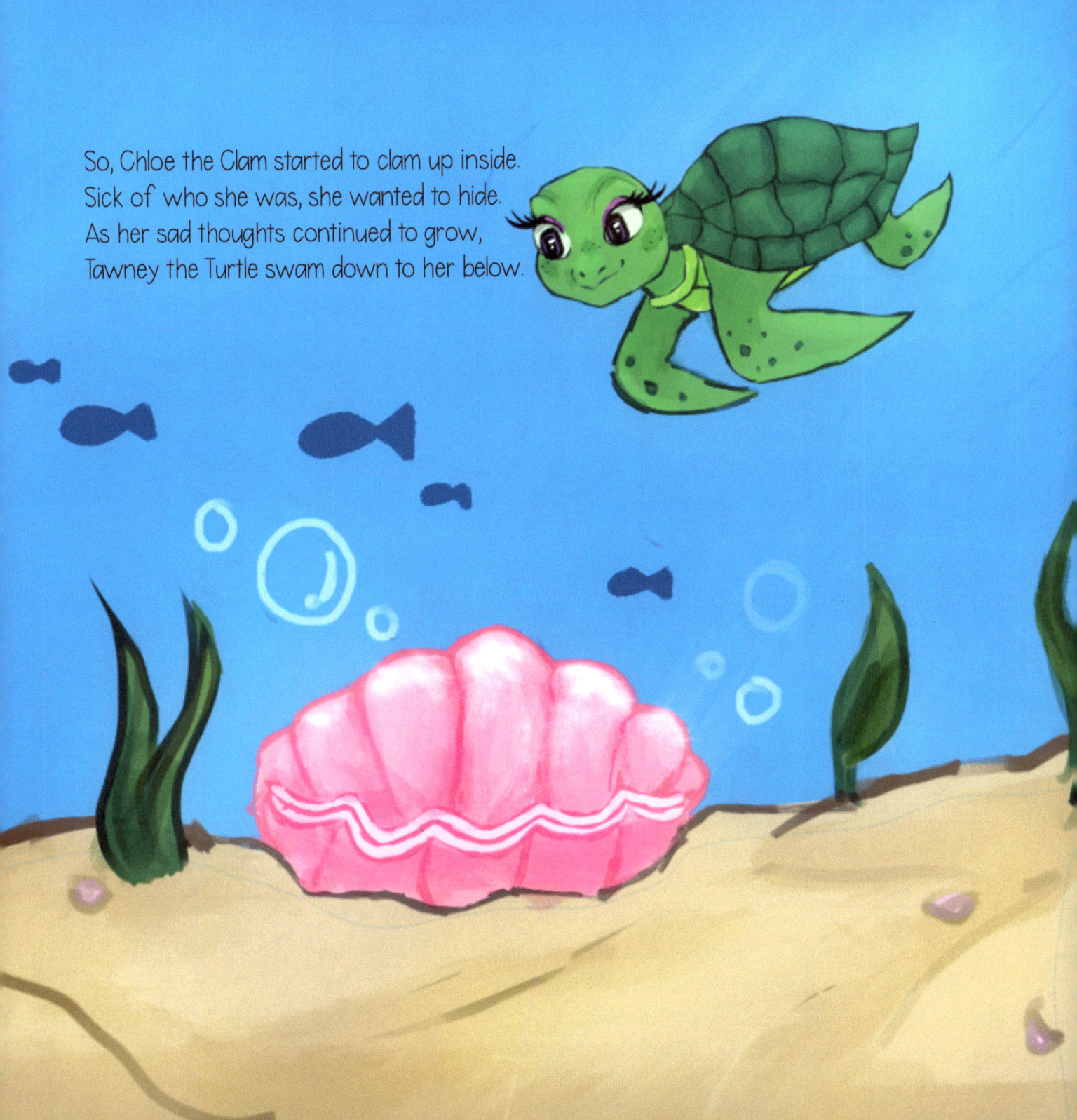

So, Chloe the Clam started to clam up inside.
Sick of who she was, she wanted to hide.
As her sad thoughts continued to grow,
Tawney the Turtle swam down to her below.

"Good Morning, Chloe!" she said with a smile.
"What's been going on? I haven't seen you in awhile!"
"Oh, nothing really, since I'm glued to this ocean floor.
But you can go anywhere! You actually get to explore!"

Sensing Chloe's insecurity, Tawney replied with a grin,
"But Chloe, don't you know, the sea is so big, it can be hard to fit in."
"You lay here in peace and friends come to see you!
You don't have to surface every five hours for air like I do!"
"You also feel safe tucked there in your shell.
Sea Turtles like me can't do that when we don't feel so well."

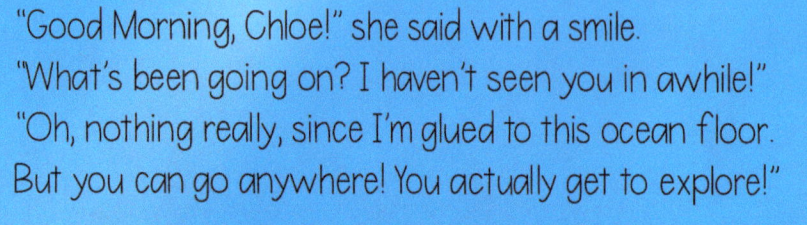

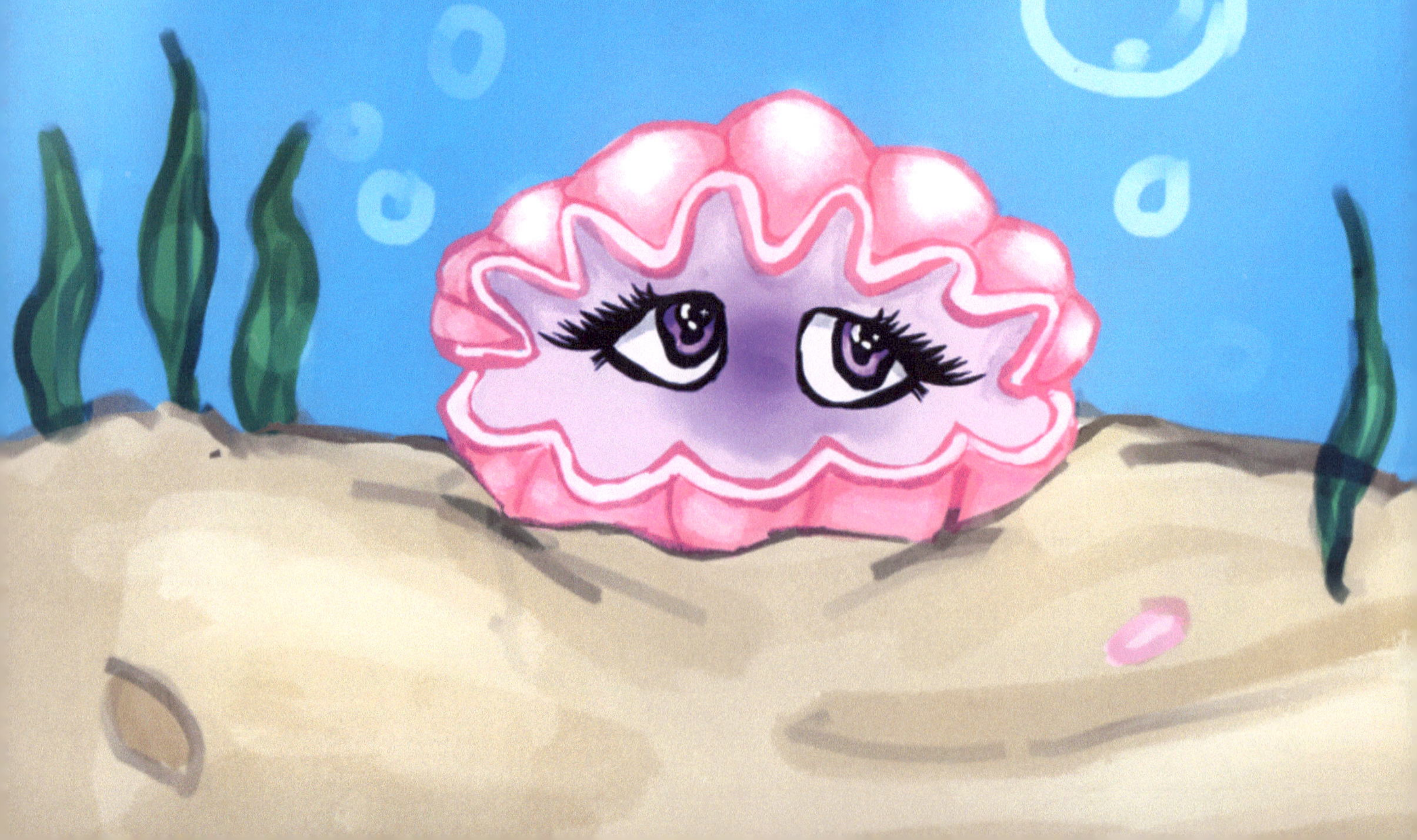

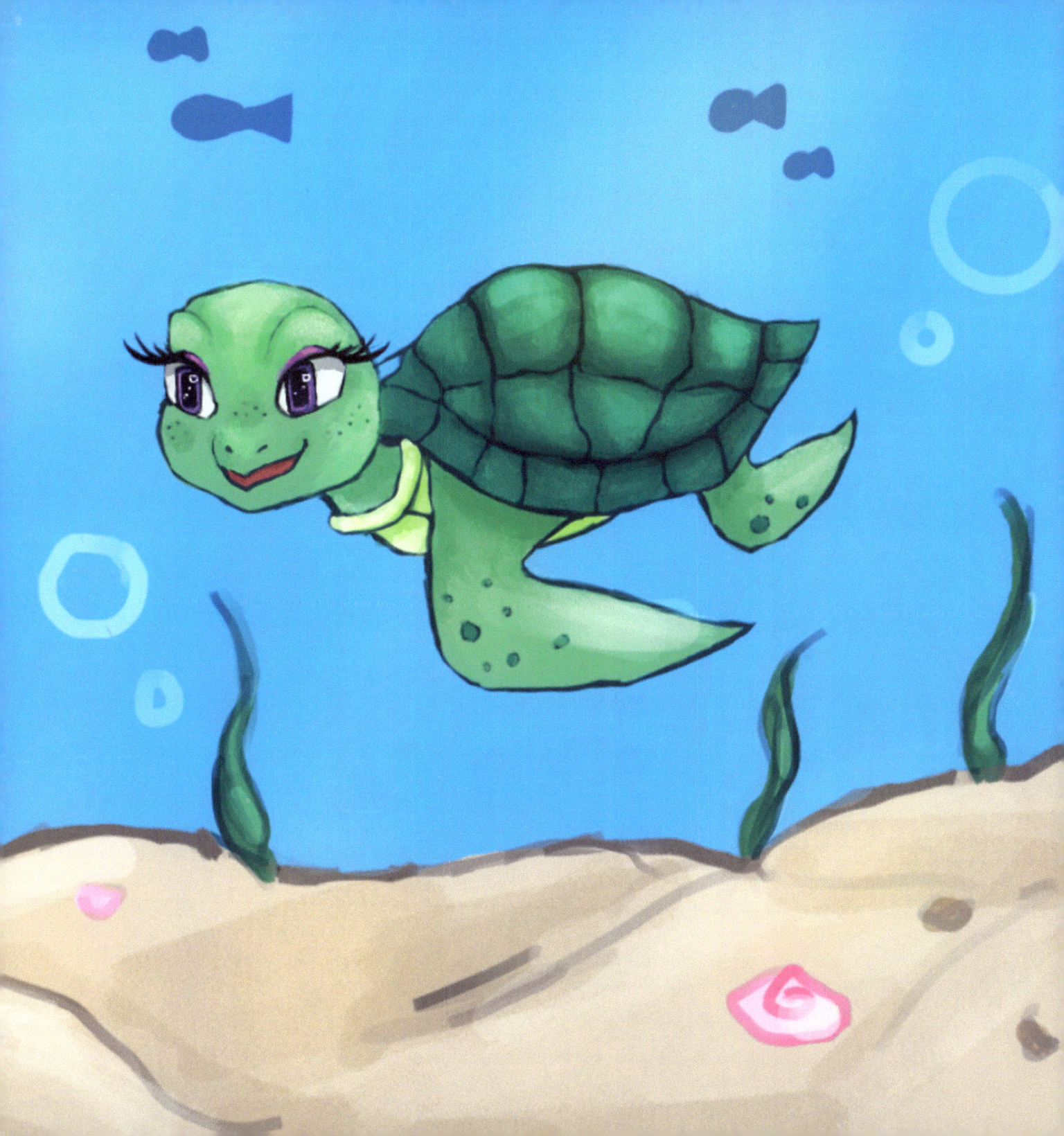

Chloe looked up at Tawney with wide big eyes.
"I am so sorry Tawney, I didn't realize!"
"It just seems so amazing to glide through the sea!
I didn't realize you might have problems too, that you could be like me!"

"Thank you for taking time to see me today,"
said Chloe to her friend Tawney, as she swam away.
But as the Sea Turtle left, Chloe sat alone again.
Her thoughts began to wander, an unknown feeling began.
I guess Tawney was right - I can protect myself inside.
I can be seen by everyone, or by no one when I need to hide.

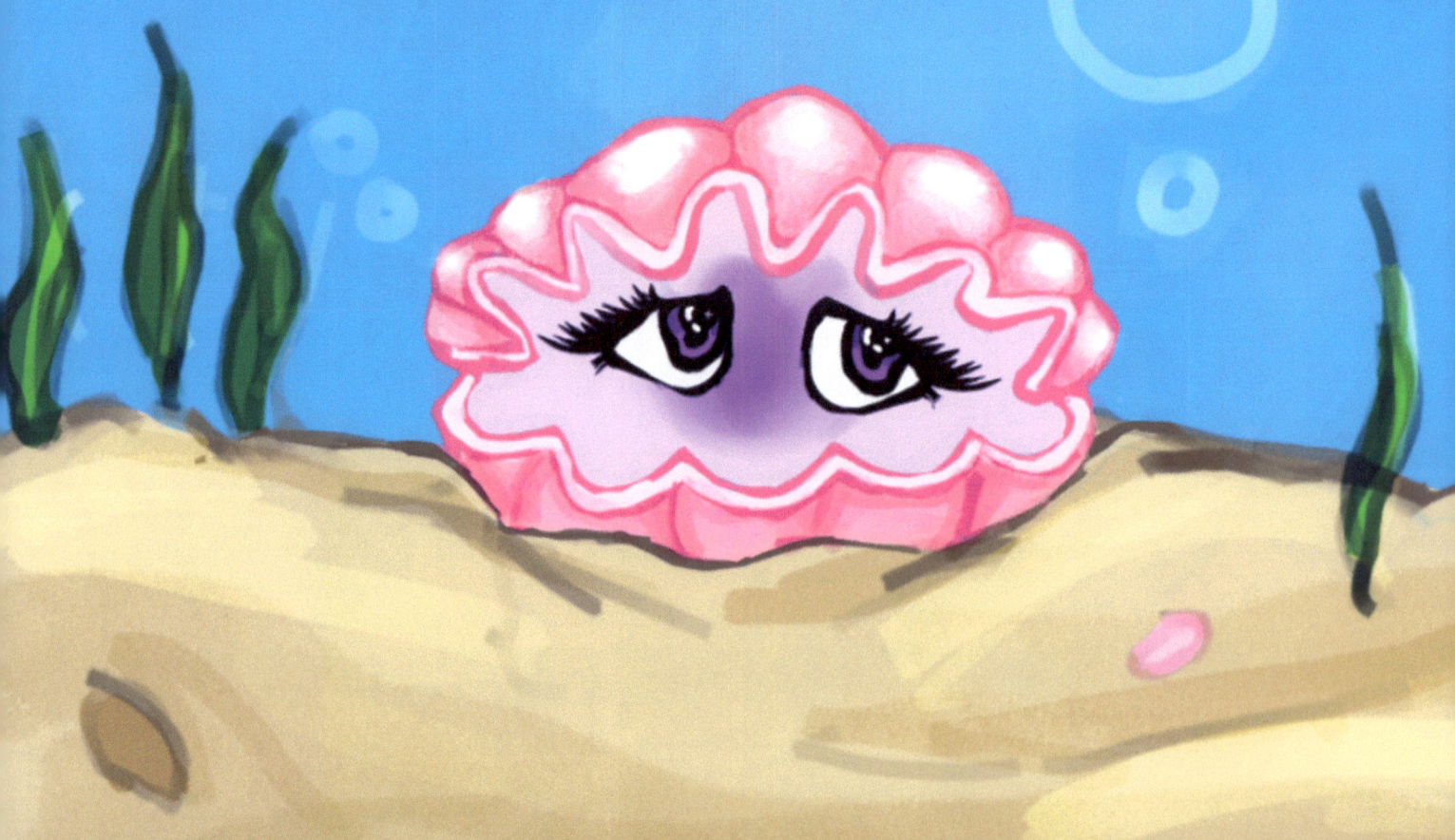

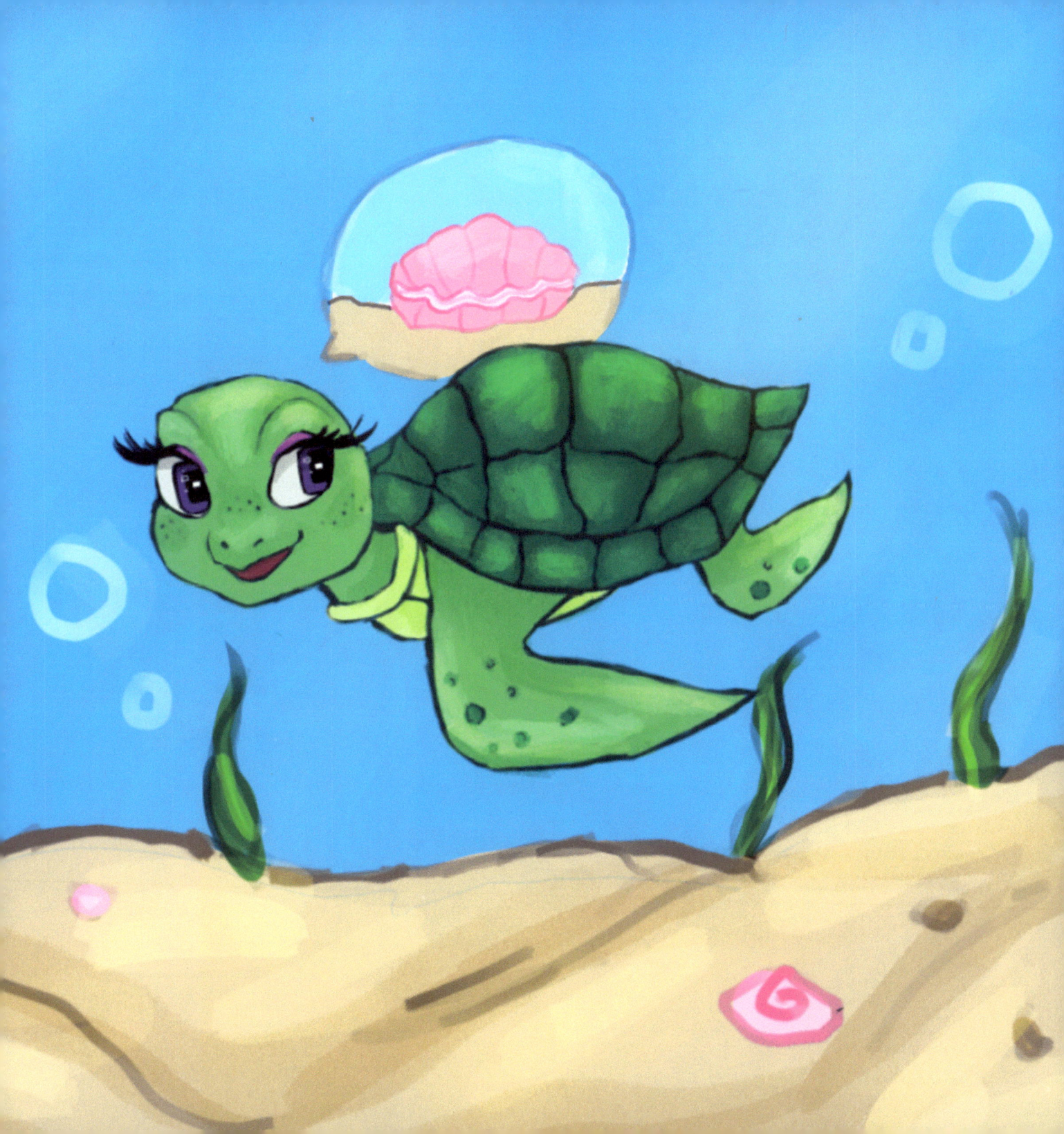

Then just as she was closing her shell,
she heard another voice she knew so well.
Sally the Seahorse called to Chloe in her high sing-song voice.
"Chloe my dear, open back up!" and knowing Ms. Sally, Chloe
felt she had no choice.

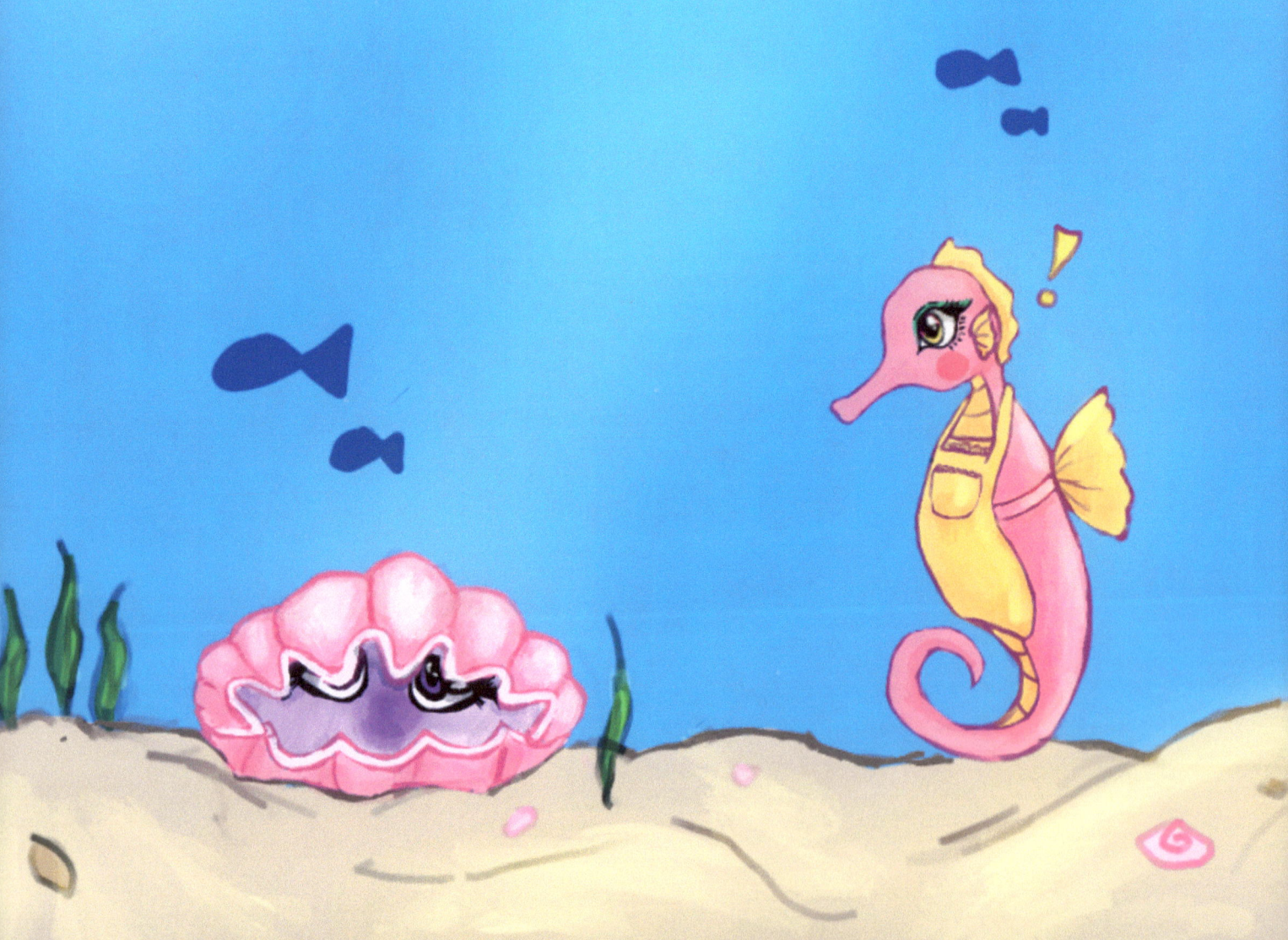

" Hello Ms. Sally, How is your day?" Unsure of what Ms. Sally needed,
this was all she could think of to say.
"Oh, Chloe my darling, as you have just been sitting here,
have you seen my darling Stan? I was supposed to meet him near!"
"Um, no Ms. Sally I haven't seen him swimming along this way."
The words came out more sassy than how she meant to say.
" Oh, Sorry I just lay here with nothing else to do,
not swimming around with my life long mate, like you
get to do!"

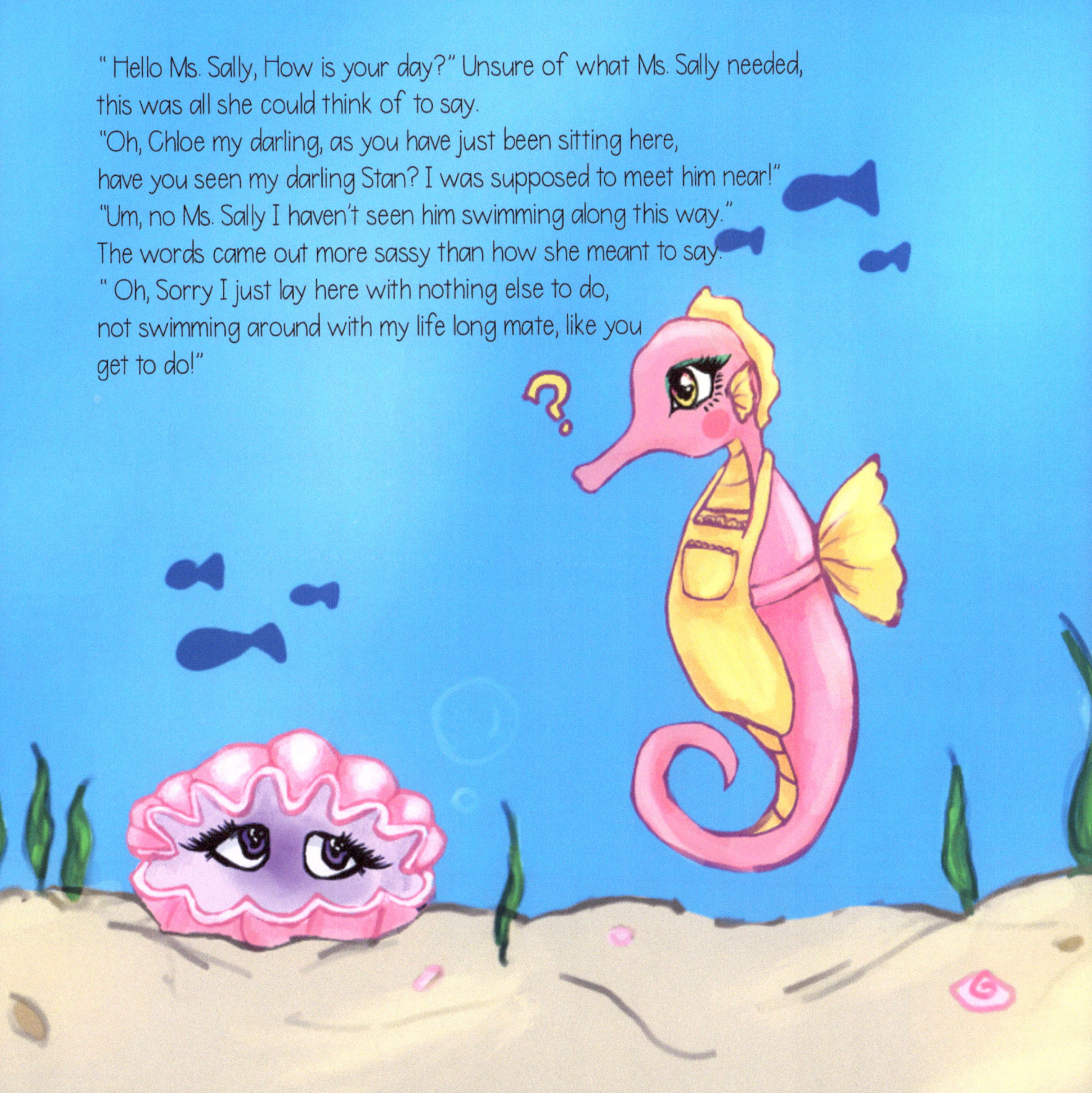

"Did I say something to you to hurt you Chloe?" Ms. Sally's sing-song voice said with concern.

Chloe suddenly felt guilty and her eyes began to burn.

"I am sorry Ms. Sally. I guess I got jealous of you and your mate. You get each other for life, and what is my fate?"

"To be here alone forever and ever with nobody to share my life with on this ocean floor? Who would want to sit here all day, with life being such a bore?"

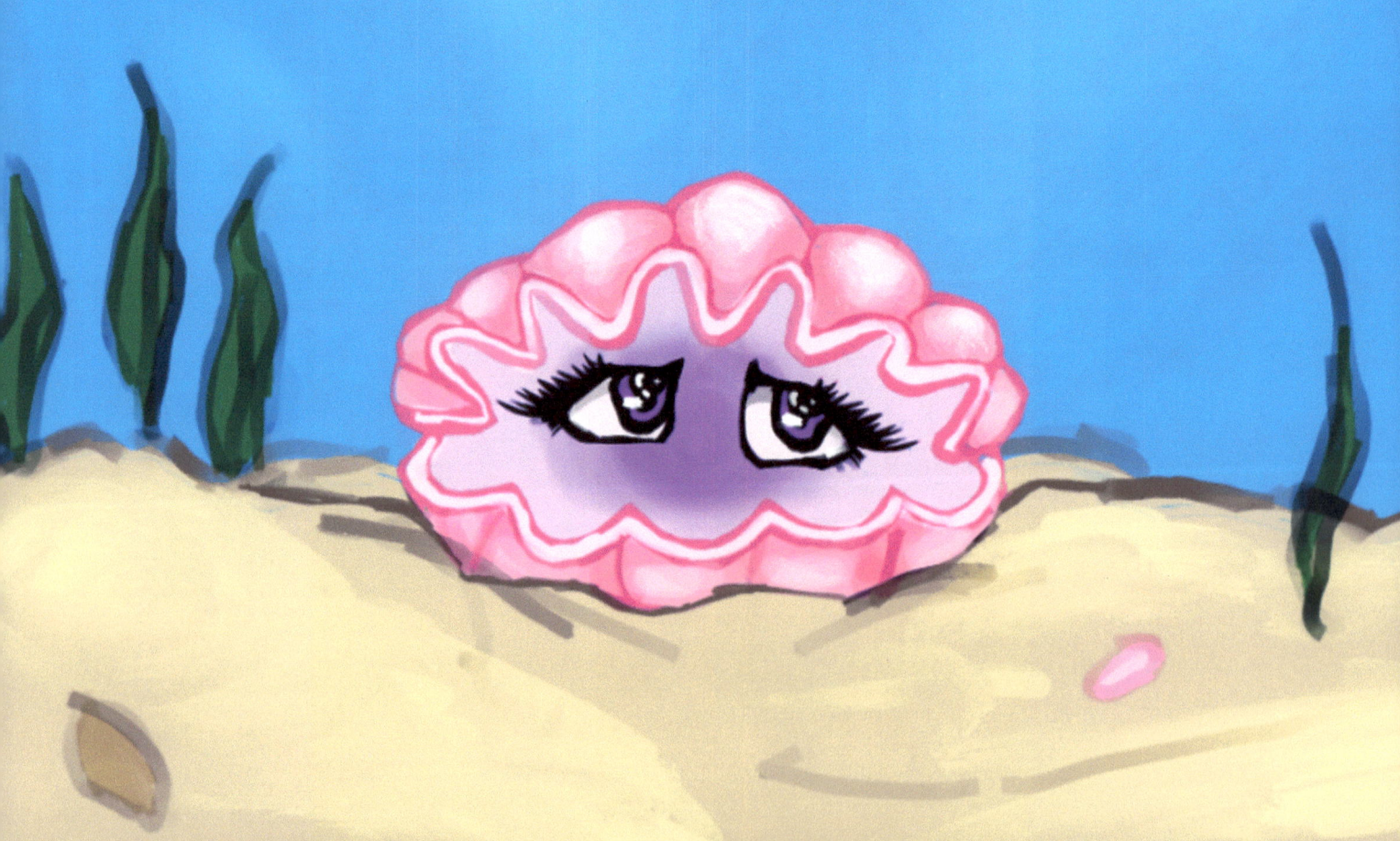

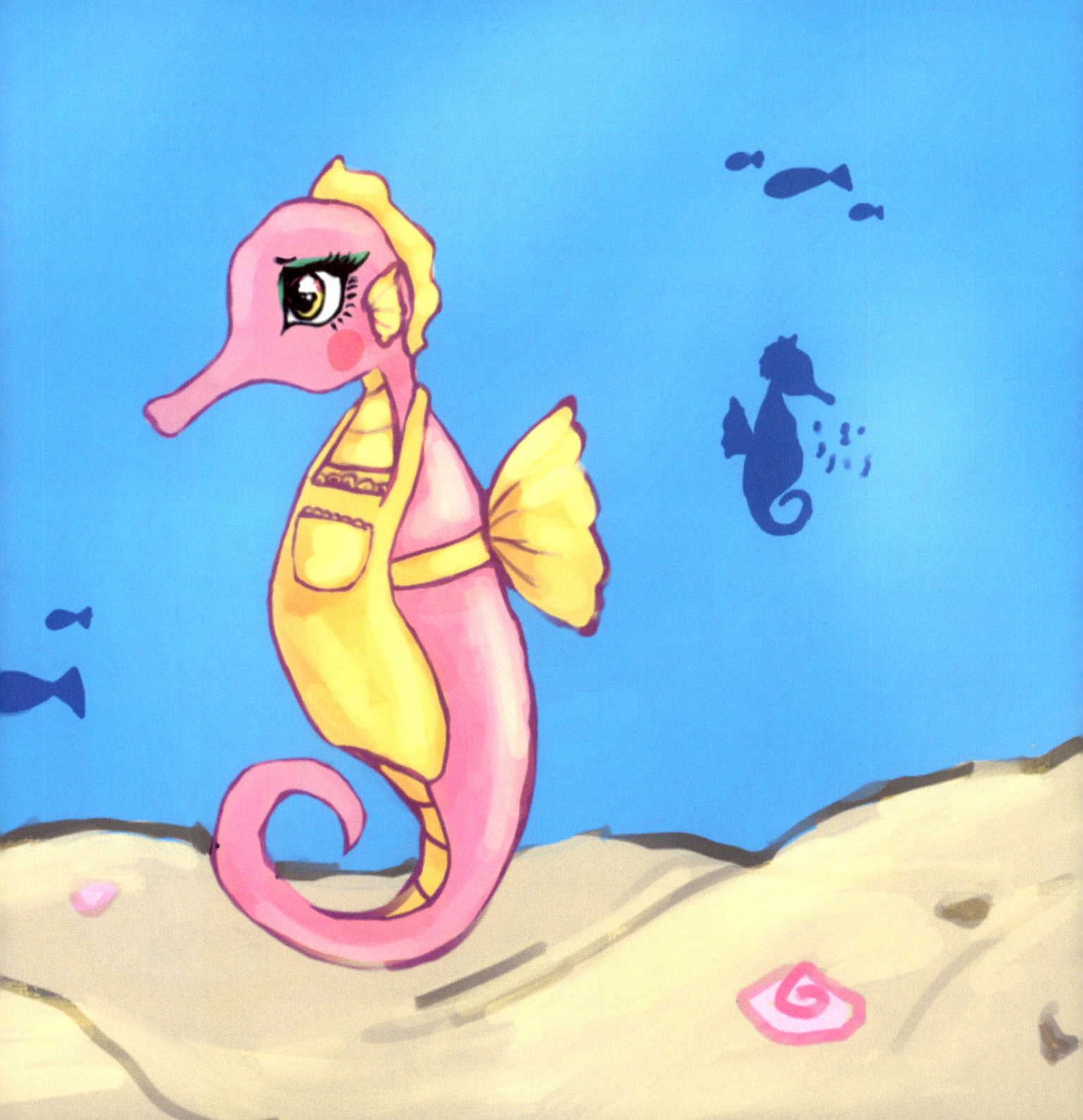

Ms. Sally looked at Chloe with one eye, and then with the other.
"Oh Darling Chloe, yes I am lucky to have Stan, of course.
But did you know I made 2000 fry to hand off to that seahorse?"
"I am tired and worn out, I would love to take your place!
You get to relax, take time for yourself, and do things at your own pace!"
"I give and I give and sometimes it doesn't feel like enough!
Sorry, Chloe dear. I shouldn't burden you with all that stuff."

"No!" Chloe said, raising her voice up loud.
"You have so much to be grateful for, you should be so proud!
You need to remember that as you are being Seahorse of the year.
Still take time for yourself even with Stan and 2000 kids near!"
"Sally!" Stan called from the coral across the way.
"I think the kids are coming!" So, off Sally went to
save the day.

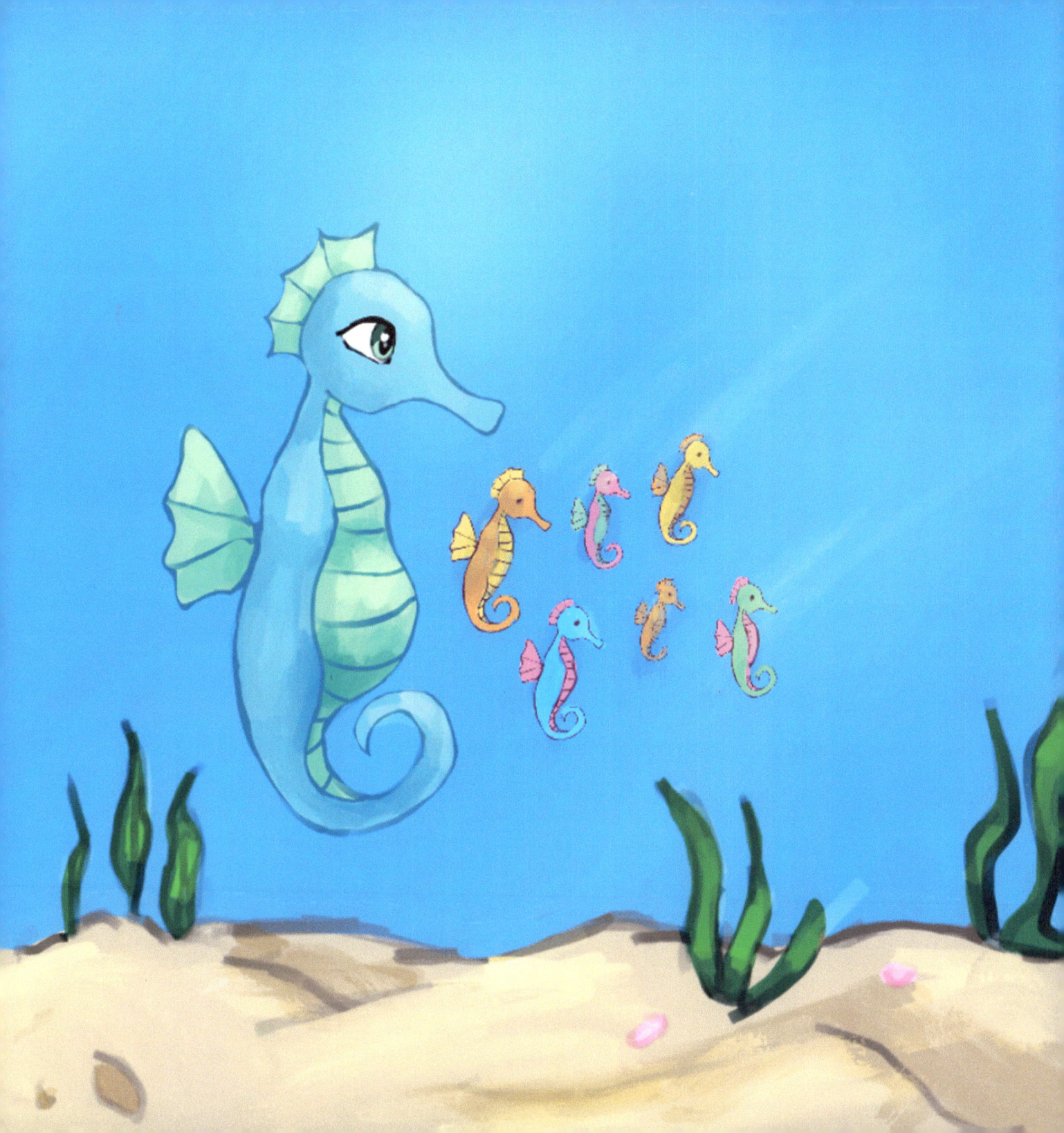

Chloe thought to herself, my time will come someday.
If not, at least my own company is great anyway.
Feeling more positive, Chloe looked back up at the sea,
but then a puddle of doubt crept back in instantly!

There they were above her, swimming together in a row.
The gorgeous parrot fish flashed the colors of the rainbow.
They were stunning and beautiful to everyone who they swam by.
"I wish others thought I was beautiful." Chloe said with a sigh.
"Oh hey Reina, Rupert, Regina, and Ray."
Chloe said as they descended to the sand where she lay.
"Hey Chlo." They said together like cool popular fish do.
"What's going on down here, have you seen anything new?

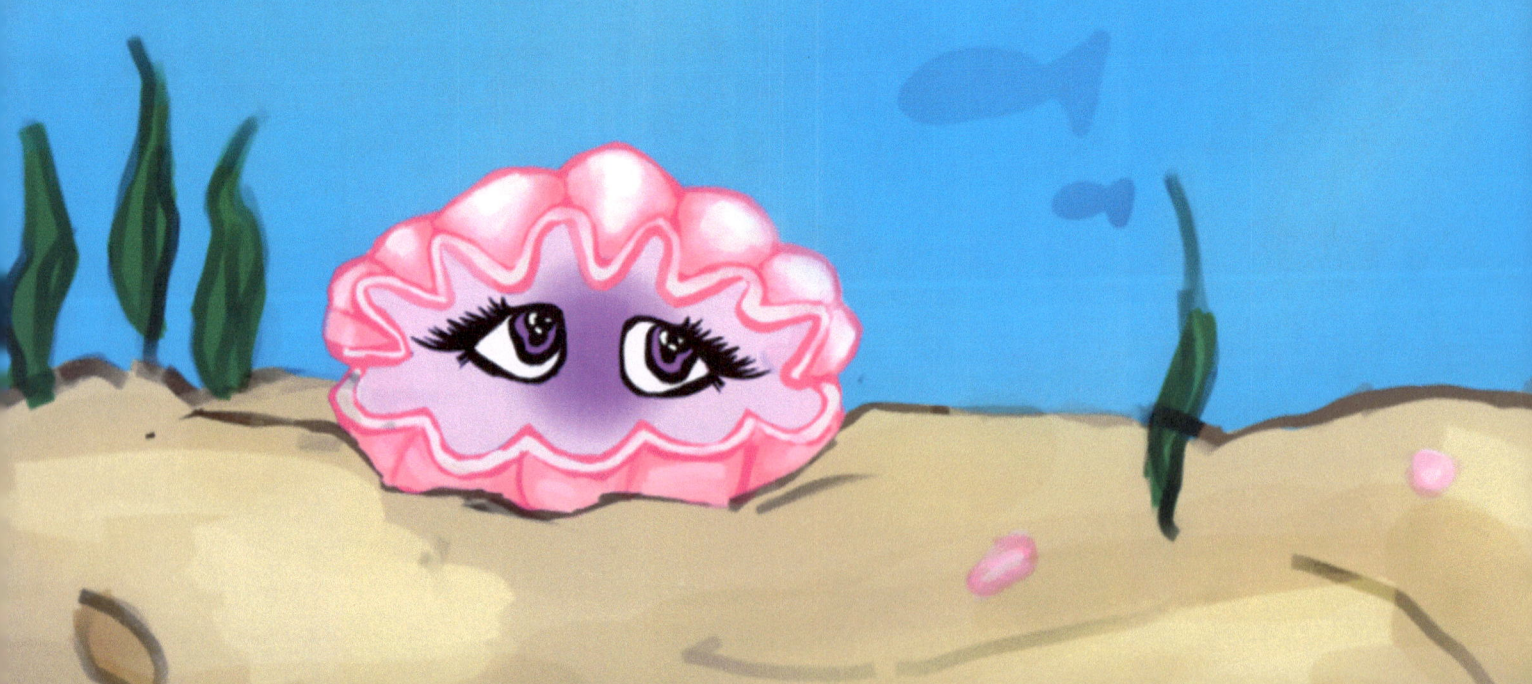

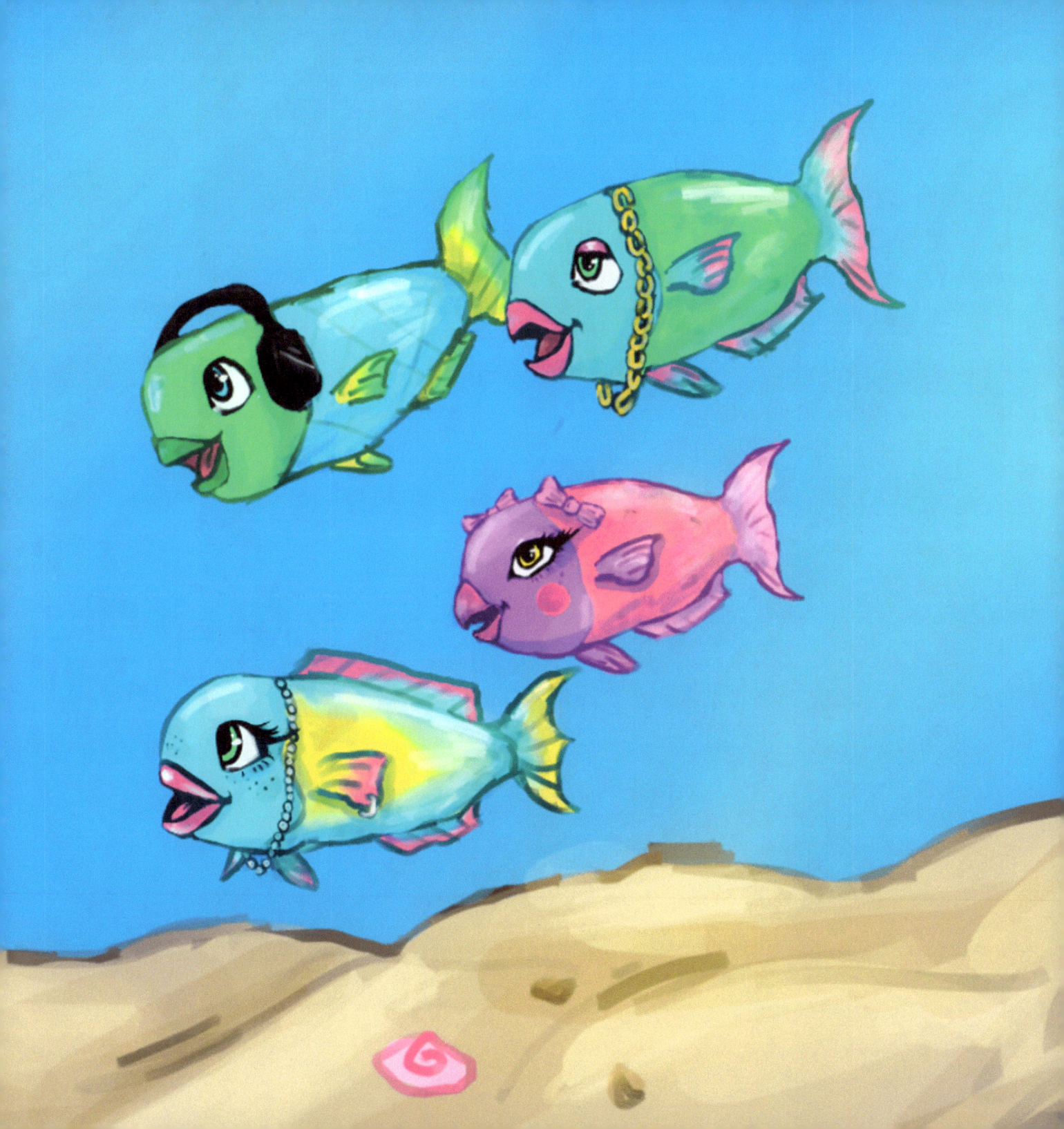

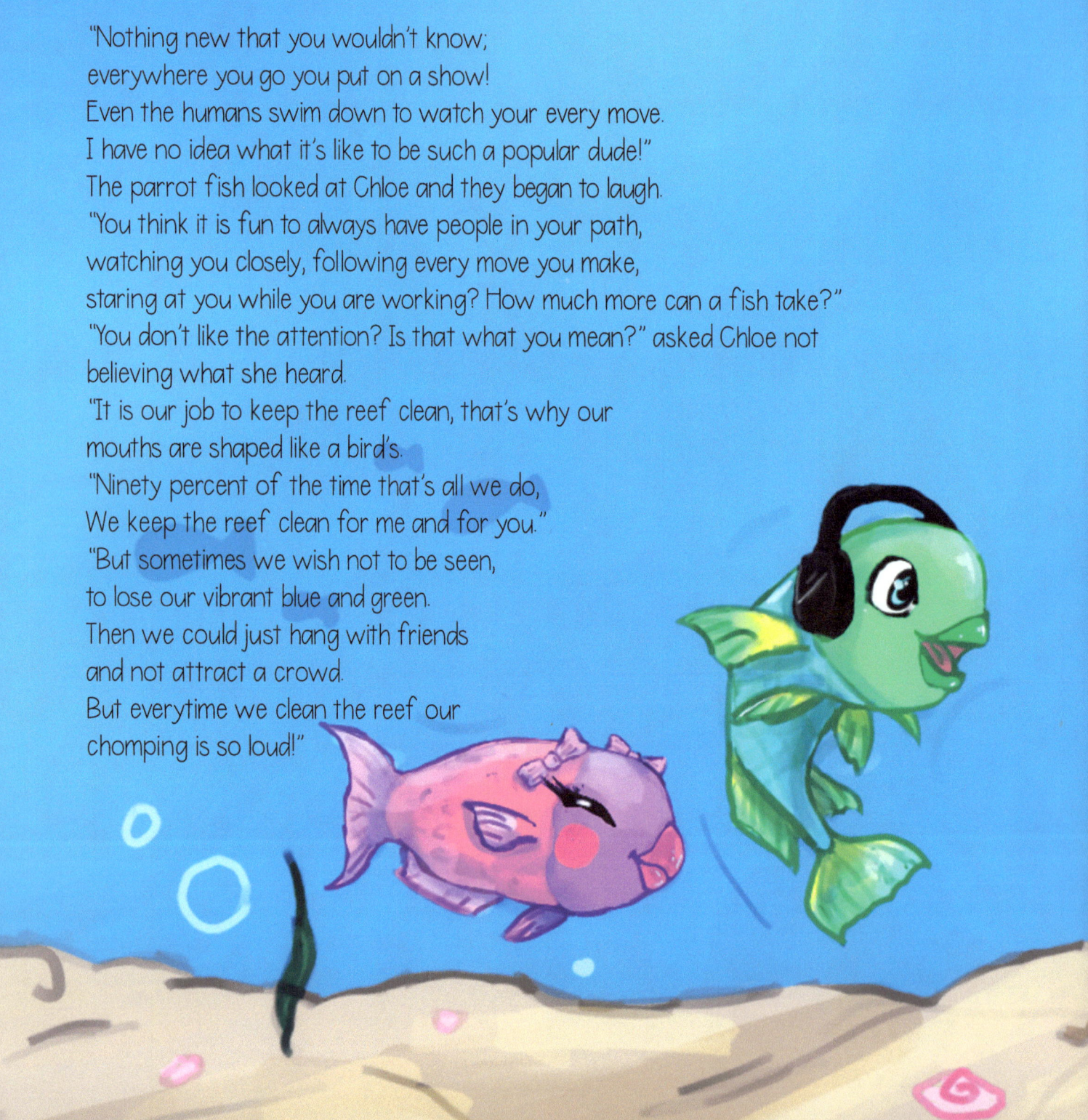

"Nothing new that you wouldn't know;
everywhere you go you put on a show!
Even the humans swim down to watch your every move.
I have no idea what it's like to be such a popular dude!"
The parrot fish looked at Chloe and they began to laugh.
"You think it is fun to always have people in your path,
watching you closely, following every move you make,
staring at you while you are working? How much more can a fish take?"
"You don't like the attention? Is that what you mean?" asked Chloe not
believing what she heard.
"It is our job to keep the reef clean, that's why our
mouths are shaped like a bird's.
"Ninety percent of the time that's all we do,
We keep the reef clean for me and for you."
"But sometimes we wish not to be seen,
to lose our vibrant blue and green.
Then we could just hang with friends
and not attract a crowd.
But everytime we clean the reef our
chomping is so loud!"

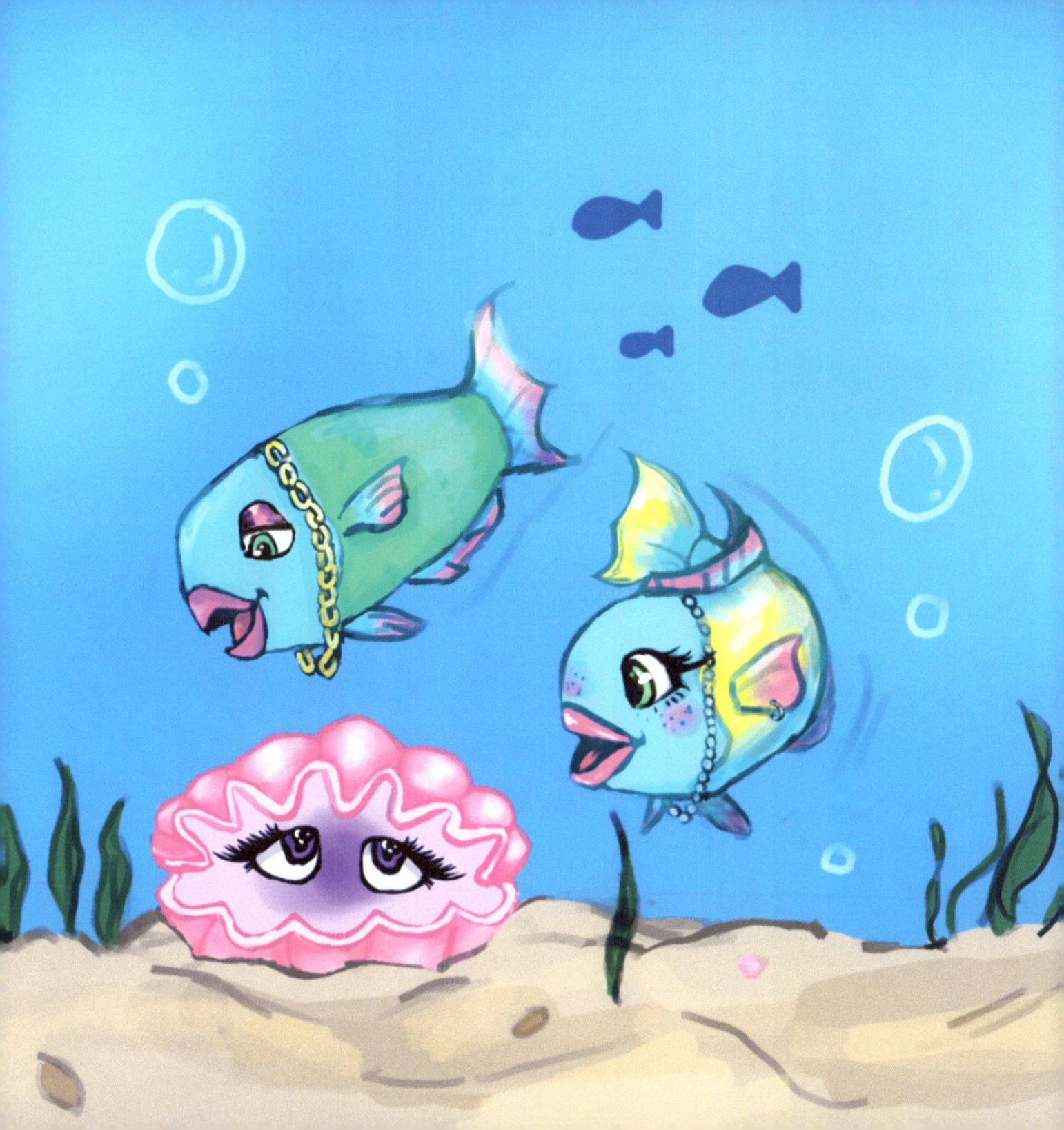

"So let me get this straight you gorgeous, awesome fish.
You don't think yourselves amazing and can do whatever you wish?
You don't think, "WOW! Everyone look at me?"
Because clearly you are some of the most beautiful fish in the sea."

"Being unique in your own way is really what beauty is all about."
Reina said to the Clam. "I try to look at the beauty in others
and be happy with who I am.
"Look at you Chlo, your eyes shine so bright
And your shell seems iridescent sparkling in the light.
You are beautiful on the inside and on the out.
Isn't that what being a good creature is all about?"

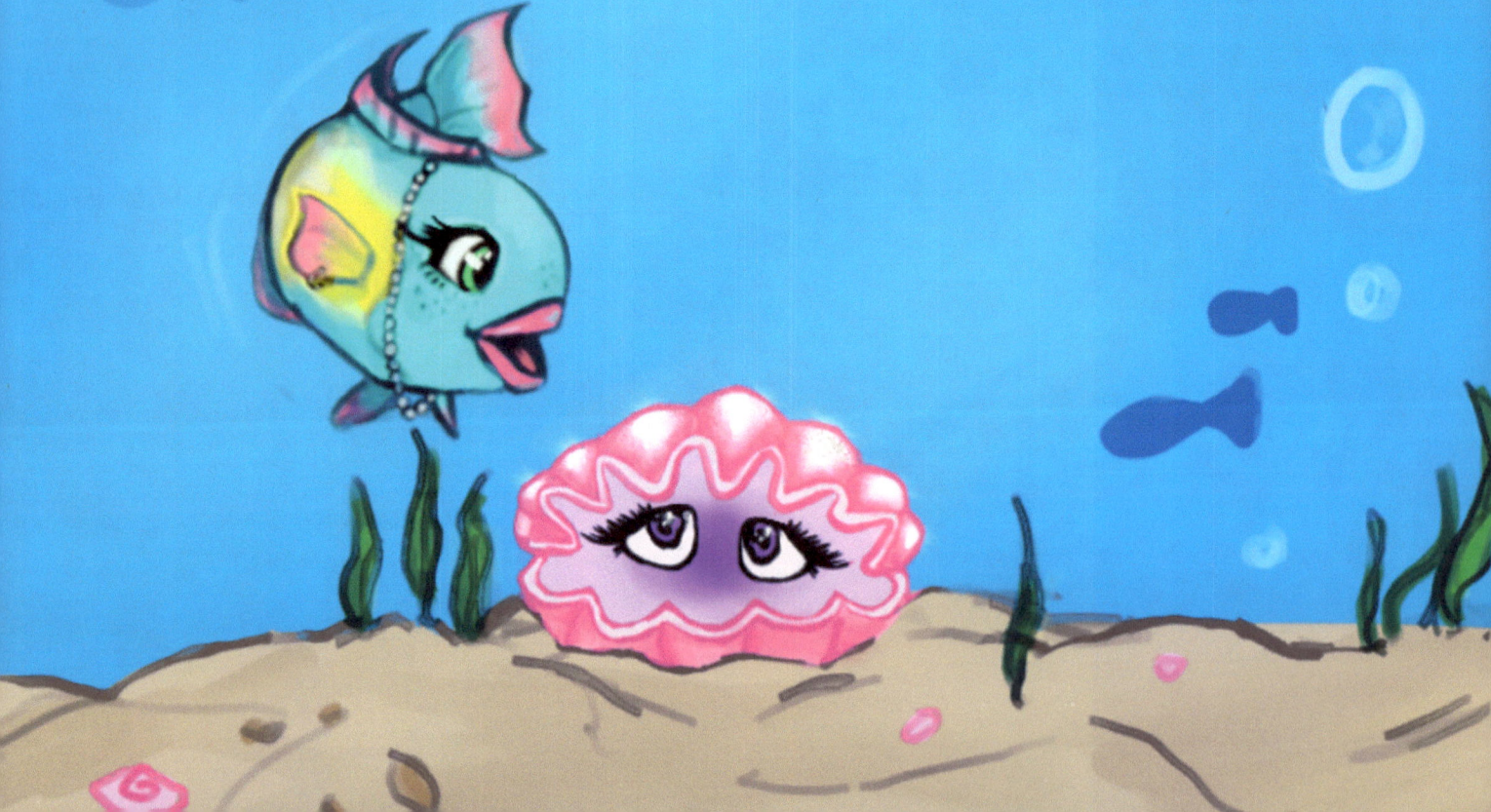

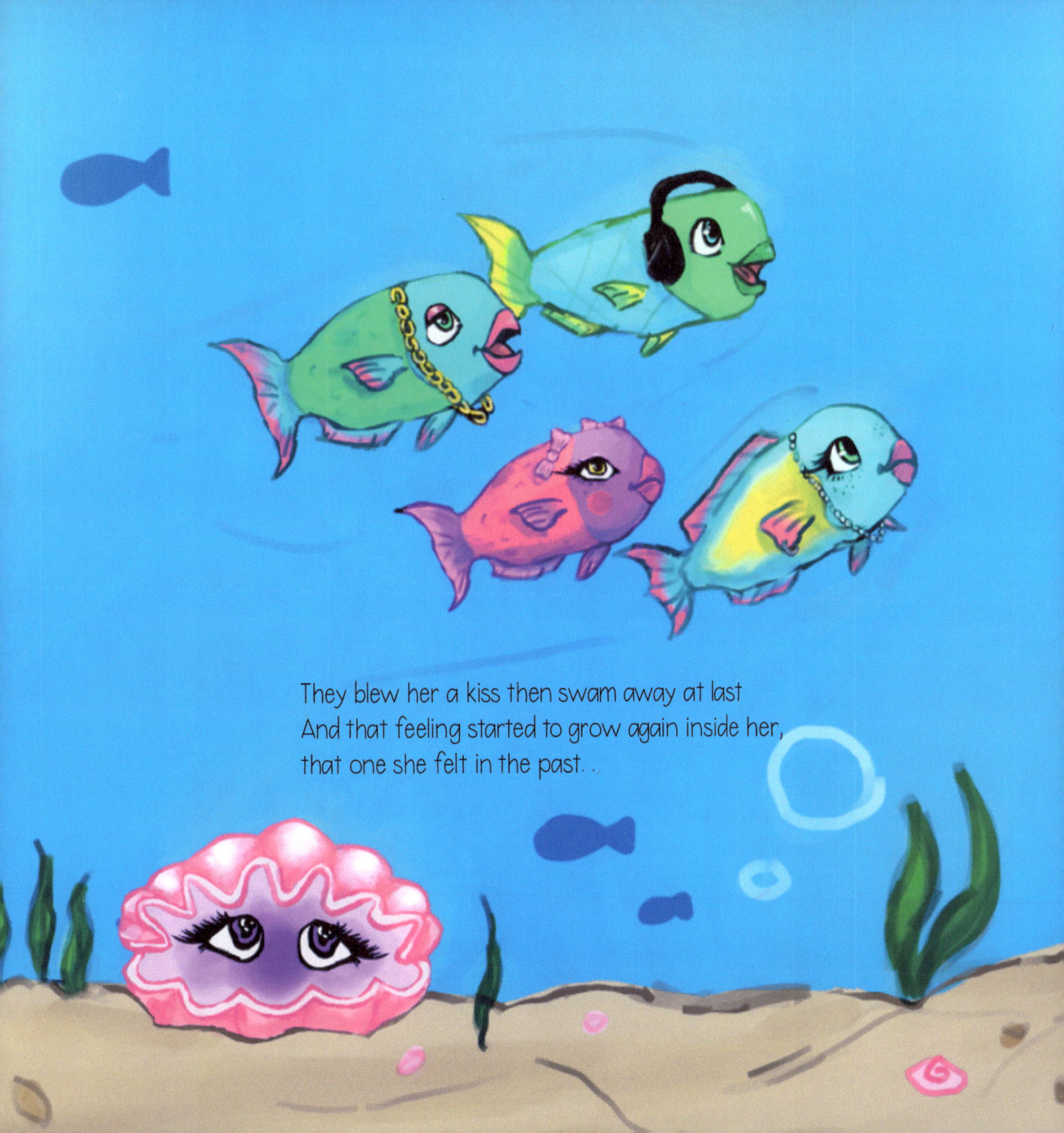

They blew her a kiss then swam away at last
And that feeling started to grow again inside her,
that one she felt in the past. . .

It was vague at first, What was she feeling inside?
Was that warm feeling, something like pride?
Suddenly a shadow emerged looming over the Clam, putting her in the dark.
At first, she was frightened until she realized it was just the Great White Shark Mark!
"Mark!" she yelped. "You gave me such a fright!"
Saddened he said "Yeah, that's about right."
"Mark, what's going on? Why do you look so sad?"
"Well everyone thinks I'm some monster and that makes me mad!
"I didn't ask to have skin six inches deep!
To have a jaw that disconnects and have rows of sharp teeth!
It's not like I want everyone to scurry when I swim on the scene!
I guess I don't like the reputation of being so mean."

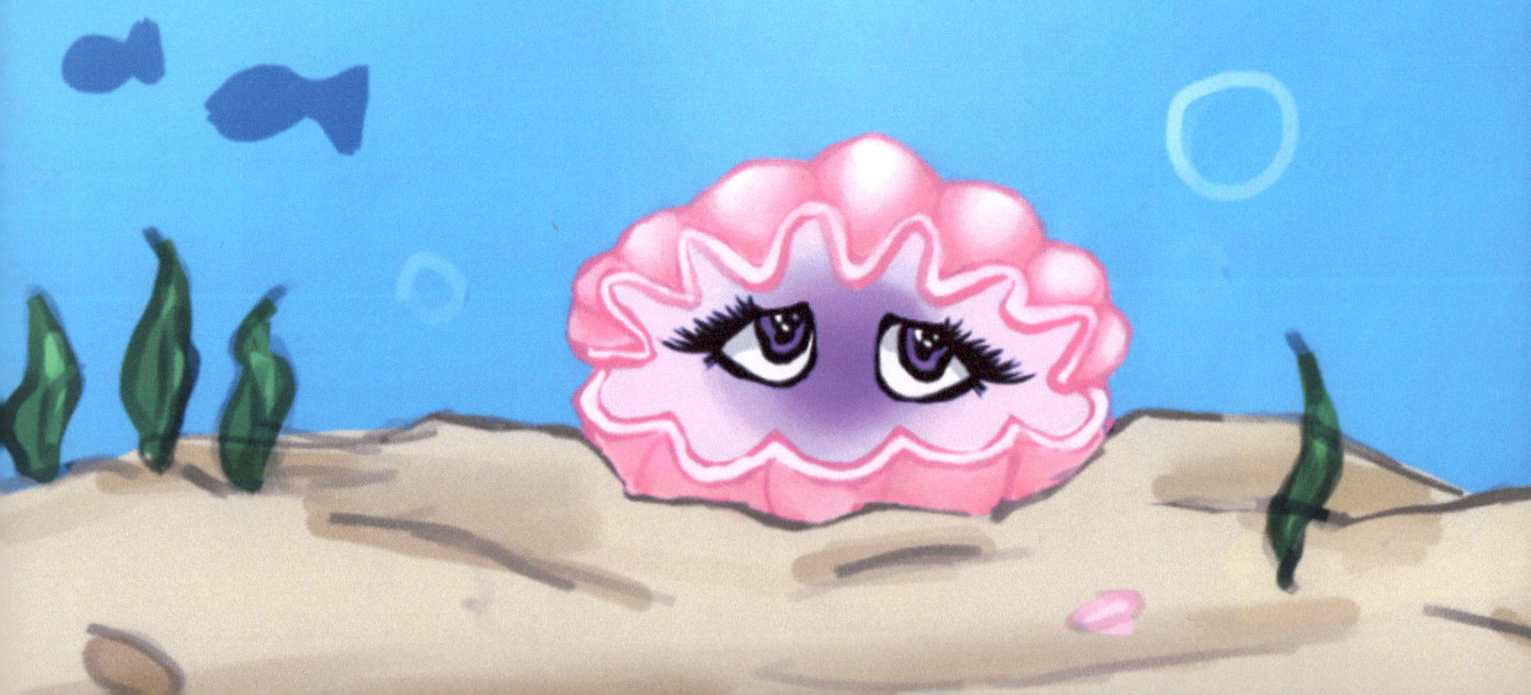

"Mark my shark, Chloe started to chide.
"Listen here buddy. That's not who you are on the inside!
I know you mind your own business unless someone gets in your way,
and you don't really hunt humans… that's just something people say!"

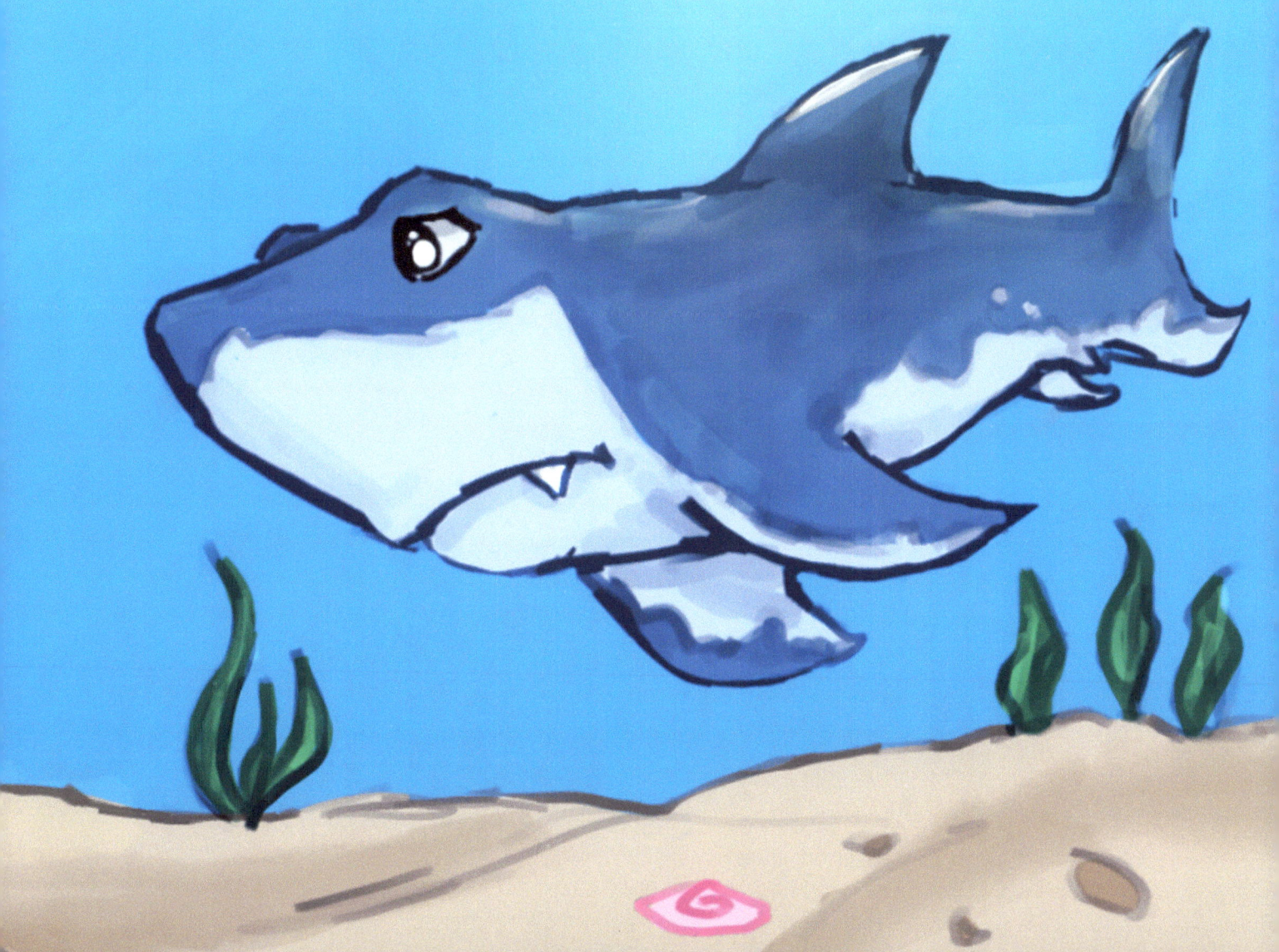

"Sometimes I am grumpy because I don't sleep at night.
I have to always be swimming in order for me to breathe right.
I can only swim forward, which makes me think I am doing something wrong,
and no one wants a toothy shark around so I feel like I don't always belong."

"Today," explained Chloe. "I have learned a few valuable truths from our friends
here in the sea. Everyone has problems, just like you and me.
We may think their lives are better and from the surface it may seem so.
But everyone is just doing their best and they have shown me how to grow.
You don't need to compare your beauty,
their extensive travels, or their sense of duty.
Do not care what others think about you, or what you have to give,
or what it is you own or where it is you live.
But my friend, you and I need to love ourselves just the way we are right now.
I know it won't be easy, but I can show you how.

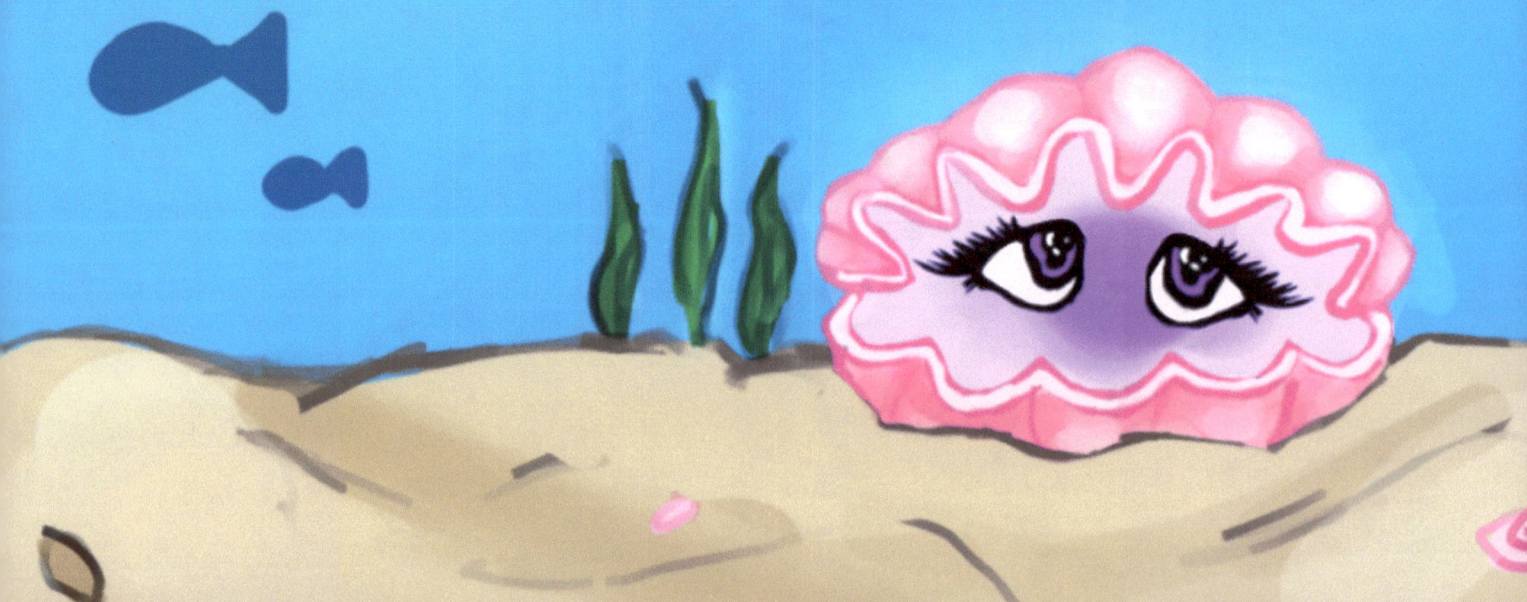

Now look at me in the eyes and repeat after me...
I am an amazing creature, a creature of the sea.
I can do anything IF I love me.

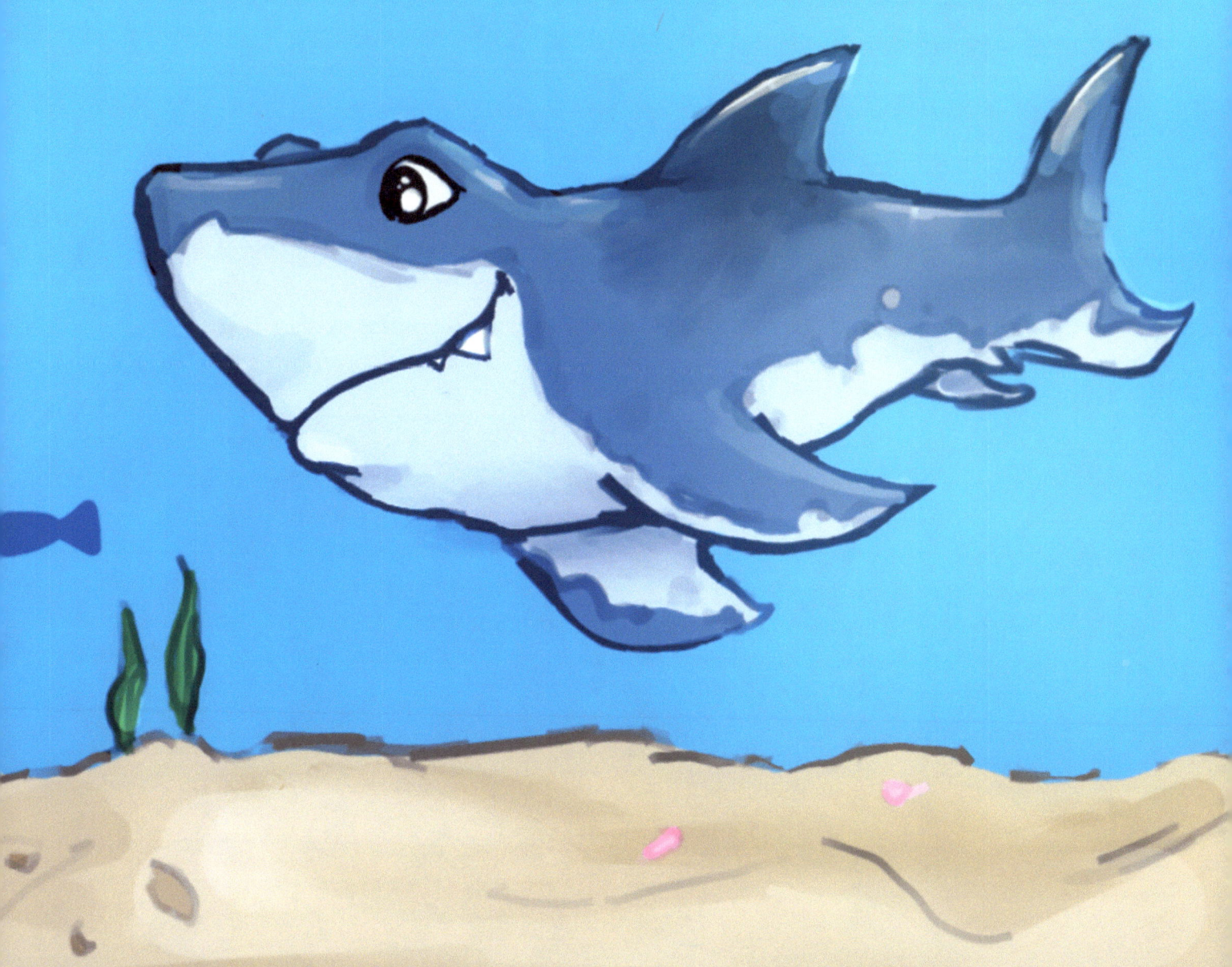

www.ingramcontent.com/pod-product-compliance
Lightning Source LLC
Chambersburg PA
CBHW041013170626
46815CB00003B/283